# American College of Surgeons
# Protocol for Cancer Surgery Documentation: Gastric Cancer

Name: ACS.CSSP.protocol.gastric.2024.v1

## What This Protocol Includes and Covers

- A synoptic operative report for gastric cancer surgery
  - Section 1: EMR Autopopulated Information
  - Section 2: Cancer-Specific Information *(required)*
  - Section 3: Additional Procedure Details
- The synoptic operative report summary template
- Knowledge Platform with explanatory notes

## American College of Surgeons Standards References

The following ACS standards references are heavily leveraged throughout the synoptic operative report and Knowledge Platform: *AJCC Cancer Staging Manual*, Eighth Edition; *Operative Standards for Cancer Surgery*, Volume 2; and Standards for *Oncology Registry Entry (STORE) 2023*.


## Authors

Ryan P. Merkow, MD, MS, FACS*; Waddah B. Al-Refaie, MBBCh, FACS*; Jeremy L. Davis, MD, FACS*; Travis Grotz, MD*; Haejin In, MD, MBA, MPH, FACS*

## Reviewers

Oliver Eng, MD, FACS†; Mitchell Posner, MD, FACS†; Suzanne C. Schiffman, MD, FACS†; Yanghee Woo, MD, FACS†; Anthony Dong Eun Yang, MD, MS, FACS†

## Contributors

Megan Beems, MD; Clifford Cho, MD, FACS; Gareth Eeson, MD, MSc; Ryan Fields, MD, FACS; Miral Sadaria Grandhi, MD; William Hawkins, MD, FACS; Gabriel Herrera-Almario, MD; Young K. Hong, MD; Paul Karanicolas, MD, PhD, FRCSC, FACS; Vladimir M. Kushnir, MD, FASGE; Shishir K. Maithel, MD, FACS; Harveshp Mogal, MD; Kerri Ohman, MD; Timothy M. Pawlik, MD, MPH, PhD, FACS, FRACS (Hon.); George A. Poultsides, MD, MS; Motaz Qadan, MD, PhD; Carl R. Schmidt, MD, FACS; Vivian E. Strong, MD, FACS; Jennifer Tseng, MD; Konstantinos Votanopoulos, MD, PhD, FACS; Sandra L. Wong, MD, MS, FACS, FASCO

**Denotes primary author. †Denotes synoptic operative report reviewer.*

# Synoptic Operative Report

**What This Synoptic Operative Report Covers and Includes**
This synoptic operative report (SOR) covers documentation for gastric cancer surgery.

The SOR includes roughly 15 fields for EMR autopopulated data, 17 fields for tumor-specific data (required), and nine fields for additional procedure data that assist with billing and regulatory and practice requirements. This SOR was designed for cases of primary gastric malignancy and not for benign disease. However, narrative text boxes may facilitate expanded use of this SOR at the user's discretion.

**How This SOR Is Organized**
*Required fields are indicated by an asterisk (*).*

## Section 1: EMR Autopopulated Information
Patient Name*
Patient ID*
Date of Surgery*
Name of Surgeon*
Name of Co-Surgeon
Name of Assistant(s)
Indication for Surgery*
Preoperative Diagnosis*
Postoperative Diagnosis*
Procedure(s) Performed*
Specimens Removed
Type of Anesthesia
Estimated Blood Loss
Drain/Implant
Additional Administrative Details

## Section 2: Tumor-Specific Information (required) *(required)*
Preoperative Histopathology*
Preoperative Tumor Location*
Molecular Markers*
Diagnostic Laparoscopy on Date Prior to Index Operation*
Intent of Surgery*
Surgery Type*
Preoperative Therapy*
Intraoperative Primary Tumor Findings, T Category*
Intraoperative Lymph Node Findings, N Category*
Interoperative Metastatic Findings, M Category*
Type of Resection*
Omentectomy*
Lymph Node Dissection*
Lymph Node Stations Harvested*
Margins*
Completeness of Gastric Resection*
Adjacent Organs Resected*

## Section 3: Additional Procedure Details

Operative Approach
Reconstruction Approach
Reconstruction Method
- Type of Esophago-jejunostomy
- Type of Gastro-jejunostomy

Management of Duodenal 'Stump'
Drains
Feeding Tube
Additional Procedures
Additional Surgical Variables
Intraoperative Complications

### Instructions

This report is intended for documentation at the completion of each surgical procedure.

Instructions are provided for each data field.

Explanatory notes provide reference material for each data field.

Narrative boxes are available in all sections of the SOR to allow the addition of provider-specific information as needed.

Completing all applicable data fields in the SOR will generate an SOR summary that is compliant with multiple regulatory requirements.

- **Section 1 Instructions:** You are being asked to review all the data fields in Section 1 as the information is autopopulated from the EMR and should be checked for accuracy. Please make corrections as needed and be sure to complete required fields. Throughout the tool, required fields are marked with an asterisk (*) and represent best practice.
- **Section 2 Instructions:** You are asked to complete all data fields in this section (Tumor-Specific Information) because they are required as part of best practice.
- **Section 3 Instructions:** You are not required to complete these data fields, but the additional surgical data elements included in this section (Additional Procedure Details) will support diverse coding, regulatory, and practice needs.

---

## Section 1: EMR Autopopulated Information (Note A)

The following fields are standardized across all CSSP SORs.
Patient Name*
Patient ID*
Date of Surgery*
Name of Surgeon*
Name of Co-Surgeon
Name of Assistant(s)
Indication for Surgery*
Preoperative Diagnosis*
Postoperative Diagnosis*
Procedure(s) Performed*
Specimens Removed
Type of Anesthesia
Estimated Blood Loss
Drain/Implant
Additional Administrative Details

 

## Section 2: Tumor-Specific Information (Note B)

### Preoperative Assessment

*** Preoperative Histopathology** (Note C)
Has the preoperative diagnosis been confirmed by histopathology? Select single best answer.
__ Yes
__ No

*** Preoperative Tumor Location** (Note D)
Select all that apply.
__ Cardia (Siewert Type III)
__ Fundus of stomach
__ Body of stomach
__ Gastric antrum
__ Pylorus
__ Lesser curvature of stomach
__ Greater curvature of stomach
__ Other [Narrative] (eg. Linitus plastica, Multipled tumors, etc.)

*** Molecular Markers** (Note E)
Select all that apply.
__ None
__ HER2
    __Score 0
    __ 1+
    __ 2+
    __ 3+
    __ FISH neg
    __ FISH pos
__ Microsatellite instability
    __ MMR intact
    __ MMR Deficient
    __ PCR
        __ Stable
        __ Unstable
__ CPS score/PD-L1 status [*Narrative Box*]
__ Other—Specify [*Narrative Box*]

*** Diagnostic Laparoscopy on Date Prior to Index Operation** (Note F)
Select single best answer.
__ No *[Narrative Box]*
__ Yes *[Narrative Box]*

*** Intent of Surgery** (Note G)
Was the current operation performed for curative intent? Select single best answer.
__ Yes
__ No
    *If no:*
    Select single best answer.
    __ Diagnostic intent [*Narrative Box*]
    __ Staging intent [*Narrative Box*]
    __ Palliative intent [*Narrative Box*]

 

*** Surgery Type** (Note H)
Select single best answer.
__ Elective
__ Urgent/Emergent [*Narrative Box*]

*** Preoperative Therapy** (Note I)
Select all that apply.
__ None
__ Systemic therapy (including chemotherapy, targeted therapy, immunotherapy, endocrine [hormonal] therapy, etc.) [Narrative Box]
__ Radiation therapy (including chemoradiation)
__ Other/Comments [*Narrative Box*]

## Intraoperative Findings

*** Intraoperative Primary Tumor Findings, T Category** (Note J)
Select single best answer.
__ Primary tumor does not appear to invade the serosa (visceral peritoneum) or adjacent structures (T1/T2/T3)
__ Primary tumor appears to invade the serosa (visceral peritoneum) or adjacent structures (T4)
  *[If "Primary tumor appears to invade the serosa (visceral peritoneum) or adjacent structures (T4))" is selected, display the following:]*
  Select all that apply.
  __ Tumor invades the serosa (visceral peritoneum) (T4a)
  __ Tumor invades adjacent structures/organs (T4b) [Narrative Box]
__ Primary tumor cannot be assessed (TX)

*** Intraoperative Lymph Node Findings, N Category** (Note K)
Select single best answer.
__ No suspected adenopathy (N0)
__ Suspected regional adenopathy (N1-N3)
  *[If "Suspected regional adenopathy (N1-N3)" is selected, display the following:]*
  Select single best answer.
  __ Completely resected
  __ Not completely resected [*Narrative Box*]
__ Regional lymph nodes cannot be assessed (NX)

*** Interoperative Metastatic Findings, M Category** (Note L)
Select single best answer.
__ No suspected distant metastasis (M0)
__ Suspected distant metastasis (M1)
*[If "Suspected distant metastasis (M1)" is selected, display the following:]*
Select all that apply.
  __ Peritoneum (including omentum)
  __ Liver
  __ Ovary
__ Other/Comments—Describe location [Narrative Box]

*** Type of Resection** (Note M)
Select single best answer.
__ Distal gastrectomy
__ Subtotal gastrectomy
__ Total gastrectomy
__ Proximal gastrectomy
__ Wedge resection
__ Other—Describe [*Narrative Box*]

*** Omentectomy** (Note N)
Select single best answer.
__ Total
__ Partial
__ None [Narrative]

*** Lymph Node Dissection** (Note O)
Select single best answer.
__ D0 [*Narrative Box*]
__ D1 [*Narrative Box*]
__ D2 [*Narrative Box*]
__ D3 [*Narrative box*]
__ Other—Describe [*Narrative Box*]

*** Lymph Node Stations Harvested** (Note P)
Select all that apply.
__ Right cardiac nodes (1)
__ Left cardiac nodes (2)
__ Nodes along the lesser curvature (3)
__ Nodes along the greater curvature (4)
__ Suprapyloric nodes (5)
__ Infrapyloric nodes (6)
__ Nodes along the left gastric artery (7)
__ Nodes along the common hepatic artery (8)
__ Nodes along the celiac axis (9)
__ Nodes at the splenic hilus (10)
__ Nodes along the splenic artery (distal splenic artery) (11)
__ Nodes in the hepatoduodenal ligament (12)
__ Nodes at the posterior aspect of the pancreas head (13)
__ Nodes at the root of the superior mesenteric vein (14)
__ Nodes in the mesocolon of the transverse colon (15)
__ Para-aortic lymph nodes (16)
__ Other/Comments—Describe [*Narrative Box*]

*** Margins** (Note Q)
Select all that apply.
__ Proximal
Frozen section performed?
__ Yes
Final Frozen Section Margin
__ Negative
__ Without additional resection—Describe [*Narrative Box*]
__ With additional resection—Describe [*Narrative Box*]
__ Positive—Describe [*Narrative Box*]
__ No
__ Distal
Frozen section performed?
__ Yes
Final Frozen Section Margin
__ Negative
__ Without additional resection—Describe [*Narrative Box*]
__ With additional resection—Describe [*Narrative Box*]
__ Positive—Describe [*Narrative Box*]
__ No

*** Completeness of Gastric Resection** (Note R)
Select single best answer.
__ R0/R1 (All evidence of tumor removed without visible or palpable evidence of residual in-situ tumor remaining at conclusion of case.)
__ R2 [*Narrative Box*] (Known visible or palpable tumor (whether by inspection or radiographic evidence) remains at conclusion of case.)

*** Adjacent Organs Resected** (Note S)
Select all that apply.
__ None
__ Colon
__ Pancreas
__ Spleen
__ Other [*Narrative Box*]

## Section 3: Additional Procedure Details

**Operative Approach** (Note T)
Select all that apply.
__ Open [*Narrative box*]
__ Laparoscopic [*Narrative box*]
__ Laparoscopic converted to open—Describe reason [*Narrative Box*]
__ Robot-assisted *[Narrative Box]*
__ Robot assisted converted to open—Describe reason [*Narrative Box*]

**Reconstruction Approach** (Note U)
Select all that apply.
__ Intracorporeal
__ Extracorporeal
__ Mini-laparotomy

**Reconstruction Method** (Note V)
Select all that apply.
__ Bilroth II (Loop gastrojejunostomy)
__ Roux-en-Y—Specify Roux limb length [*Narrative Box*]
__ Other—Describe [*Narrative Box*]

*[If "Total gastrectomy" was selected under* ***Type of Resection****, display the following fields:]*
**Type of Esophago-jejunostomy** (Note W)
Select all that apply.
__ Not performed
__ Stapled
__ Circular Stapler [*Narrative Box*]
__ Linear Stapler [*Narrative Box*]]
__ Handsewn [*Narrative Box*]
__ Pouch [*Narrative Box*]
__Other—Describe [*Narrative Box*]

*[If "Distal gastrectomy," "Subtotal gastrectomy," or "Other" were selected under* ***Type of Resection****, display the following fields:]*
**Type of Gastro-jejunostomy** (Note X)
Select all that apply.
__ Not performed
__ Stapled
__ Circular Stapler [*Narrative Box*]
__ Linear Stapler [*Narrative Box*]]
__ Handsewn [*Narrative Box*]
__Other—Describe [*Narrative Box*]

*[If* "Roux-en-Y" *was selected under* ***Reconstruction Method****, display the following fields:]*
**Type of Gastro-jejunostomy** (Note X)
Select all that apply.
__ Not performed
__ Stapled
__ Circular Stapler [*Narrative Box*]
__ Linear Stapler [*Narrative Box*]]
__ Handsewn [*Narrative Box*]
__Other—Describe [*Narrative Box*]

**Management of Duodenal 'Stump'** (Note Y)
Select single best answer.
__ Stapled [*Narrative Box*]
__Bioabsorbable Staple Line Reinforcement
__ Yes
__ No
Oversewn?
__ Yes
__ No
__ None
__ Other *[Narrative Box]*

**Drains** (Note Z)
Select single best answer.
__ Yes [*Narrative Box*]
__ No

**Feeding Tube** (Note AA)
Select single best answer.
__ Yes [*Narrative Box*]
__ No

**Additional Procedures** (Note AB)
Select single best answer.
__ None
__ Yes—Describe [*Narrative Box*]

**Additional Surgical Variables** (Note AC)
Select single best answer.
__ None
__ Yes—Describe [*Narrative Box*]
__ Provided elsewhere [*Narrative Box*]

**Intraoperative Complications** (Note AD)
Select single best answer.
__ None
__ Yes—Describe [*Narrative Box*]

## SOR Summary Template (Mockup)

### Gastric Cancer

**Patient Name:** *[Autopopulate from EMR]*
**Patient ID:** *[Autopopulate from EMR]*
**Date of Surgery:** *[Autopopulate from EMR]*
**Name of Surgeon:** *[Autopopulate from EMR]*
**Name of Co-Surgeon:** *[Autopopulate from EMR]*
**Name of Assistant(s):** *[Autopopulate from EMR – Nurses notes]*
**Indication for Surgery:** *[Autopopulate from EMR; **or** override with EMR pick list]*
**Preoperative Diagnosis:** *[Autopopulate from EMR; **or** override with SOR selections]*
**Postoperative Diagnosis:** *[Autopopulate from EMR; **or** override with SOR selections]*
**Procedure(s) Performed:** *[Autopopulate from EMR; **or** override with SOR selections]*
**Specimens Removed:** *[Autopopulate from EMR – Nurses notes with override capability]*
**Type of Anesthesia:** *[Autopopulate from EMR – Anesthesia with override capability]*
**Estimated Blood Loss:** *[Autopopulate from EMR – Anesthesia with override capability]*
**Drain/Implant** *[Autopopulate from EMR – Nurses notes with override capability]*
**Additional Administrative Details:** *[Autopopulate from EMR; **or** Narrative text]*

**Tumor-Specific Information**

Preoperative Assessment

*[Fill from SOR: Preoperative Histopathology]*
*[Fill from SOR: Preoperative Tumor Location]*
*[Fill from SOR: Molecular Markers]*
*[Fill from SOR: Diagnostic Laparoscopy on Date Prior to Index Operation]*
*[Fill from SOR: Intent of Surgery]*
*[Fill from SOR: Surgery Type]*
*[Fill from SOR: Preoperative Therapy]*

Intraoperative Findings

*[Fill from SOR: Intraoperative Primary Tumor Findings, T Category]*
*[Fill from SOR: Intraoperative Lymph Node Findings, N Category]*
*[Fill from SOR: Interoperative Metastatic Findings, M Category]*
*[Fill from SOR: Type of Resection]*
*[Fill from SOR: Omentectomy]*
*[Fill from SOR: Lymph Node Dissection]*
*[Fill from SOR: Lymph Node Stations Harvested]*
*[Fill from SOR: Margins]*
*[Fill from SOR: Completeness of Gastric Resection]*
*[Fill from SOR: Adjacent Organs Resected]*

**Additional Procedure Details**

*[Fill from SOR: Operative Approach]*
*[Fill from SOR: Reconstruction Approach]*
*[Fill from SOR: Reconstruction Method and if applicable Type of Esophago-jejunostomy and/or Type of Gastro-jejunostomy]*
*[Fill from SOR: Management of Duodenal 'Stump']*
*[Fill from SOR: Drains]*
*[Fill from SOR: Feeding Tube]*
*[Fill from SOR: Additional Procedures]*
*[Fill from SOR: Additional Surgical Variables]*
*[Fill from SOR: Intraoperative Complications]*

# Knowledge Platform

**Introductory Comments**
This protocol is intended to standardize documentation and communication of critical components of gastric cancer surgery. The following explanatory notes reference critical elements for cancer surgery as described in the *Operative Standards for Cancer Surgery,* Volume 2, and expert panel consensus

## Instructions

Each explanatory note is linked from a corresponding data element in the SOR above and contains additional materials and references that can be used to facilitate accurate completion of the report.

## Section 1: EMR Autopopulated Information

**Note A:** EMR Autopopulated Information

**Explanatory Comments:** The following fields are intended to be prepopulated with site-specific identifiers and information from the EMR.

Patient Name
Patient ID
Date of Surgery
Name of Surgeon
Name of Co-Surgeon
Name of Assistant(s)
Indication for Surgery
Preoperative Diagnosis
Postoperative Diagnosis
Procedure(s) Performed
Specimens Removed
Type of Anesthesia
Estimated Blood Loss
Drain/Implant
Additional Administrative Details

## Section 2: Cancer-Specific Information

**Note B:** Tumor-Specific Information

**Explanatory Comments:** This section of the SOR contains critical oncology data elements supported by evidence and best practice, as well as data fields defined by the STORE manual and submitted to hospital registries for NCDB and state registry reporting.

There are data fields in this section related to findings and/or treatments in both the preoperative and intraoperative phases of care. To complete the preoperative data fields assumes that the patient has undergone appropriate diagnostic imaging of the primary tumor, as well as the presence of regional or distant metastasis. For additional details, please refer to the *Operative Standards for Cancer Surgery,* Volume 2, pages 67–178.

 

**Note C:** Preoperative Histopathology

**Explanatory Comments:** This SOR is intended for use in all cases where there is reasonable clinical suspicion that the patient has a gastric tumor, even if the histopathology does not confirm the diagnosis preoperatively. To adjudicate any ambiguity in classification of tumors, please refer to the WHO histology classification of tumors codes listed in the *AJCC Cancer Staging Manual*, Eighth Edition, Chapter 17.

**Note D:** Preoperative Tumor Location

**Explanatory Comments:** Tumor location and/or identification of synchronous tumors is important for surgical planning and is typically determined by preoperative imaging, sometimes aided by endoscopic ultrasonography. Understanding that intraoperative findings may alter the tumor location and extent of disease, tumor location should be indicated based on preoperative imaging by selecting a single best answer for a solitary lesion or selecting all answers that apply for multiple lesions.

NCDB coding instructions for Primary Site [400] are detailed in the *STORE 2023* manual. The primary site is recorded as a "C" preceding the three-digit code number (see Table 1).

**Table 1.** Relevant NCDB Codes for Primary Site for Stomach Tumors

| NCDB Code | Definition |
|---|---|
| C160 | Cardia, esophagogastric junction |
| C161 | Fundus of stomach |
| C162 | Body of stomach |
| C163 | Gastric antrum |
| C164 | Pylorus |
| C165 | Lesser curvature of stomach, NOS |
| C166 | Greater curvature of stomach, NOS |
| C168 | Overlapping lesion of stomach |
| C169 | Stomach, NOS |

**Note E:** Molecular Markers

**Explanatory Comments:** The molecular classification of gastric cancer is important for treatment and prognostic considerations. Molecular markers with actional therapies are included for certain patients with gastric cancer. Individuals with HER2 overexpression may be eligible for trastuzumab therapy in certain cases with locally advanced, unresectable, and/or metastatic disease. Universal testing for MSI by PCR or MMR by IHC should be performed on all new gastric cancer patients. PD-L1/CPS testing may be considered in locally advanced, recurrent, or metastatic gastric cancer. The PD-L1 /CPS score is measured by the number of PD-L1 stained cells divided by the total number of cells evaluated, multiplied by 100. A specimen is considered to have PD-L1 expression if the CPS is greater than or equal to 1. If other molecular diagnostic testing was performed with significant results, please specify in the 'Other' category. For additional details, please refer to the Immunohistochemical Criterial for Scoring HER2 Express in Gastric Cancer table found in *Gastric Cancer, Version 2.2022, NCCN Clinical Practice Guidelines in Oncology*.

 

**Note F:** Diagnostic Laparoscopy on Date Prior to Index Operation

**Explanatory Comments:** Diagnostic laparoscopy should be considered to assess for intraabdominal peritoneal metastasis and perform washings to evaluate for cytology positive occult metastatic disease. Diagnostic laparoscopy with washings is recommended in all medically fit patients with potentially resectable stage cT1b or higher locoregional disease as a part of the staging workup. Patients who have undergone preoperative chemotherapy followed by the index operation will have had diagnostic laparoscopy prior to preoperative chemotherapy. For additional details, please refer to the *Operative Standards for Cancer Surgery*, Volume 2, pages 77-81.

**Note G:** Intent of Surgery

**EExplanatory Comments:** Intent should be assigned postoperatively by the operating surgeon on the basis of preoperative evaluation and intraoperative management. Intent should be documented as part of the operative report. Curative operations generally include complete resection of the primary tumor and regional lymphadenectomy for therapeutic or staging purposes. If the operation was not performed for curative intent, response options are provided for diagnostic, staging, or palliative intent along with narrative boxes to record any additional information.

**Note H:** Surgery Type

**Explanatory Comments:** For gastric cancer surgery, it is important to determine if this is an elective planned oncologic resection or if the symptoms of the gastric cancer warrant urgent or emergent surgical intervention to palliate symptoms (bleeding, perforation, or obstruction) and thus not all oncologic principles may apply. Surgery type should be assigned by the operating surgeon and documented.

**Note I:** Preoperative Therapy

**Explanatory Comments:** For gastric adenocarcinoma cT2-4 or N+, multimodality therapy should be considered according to national guidelines. There are multiple options of perioperative therapy, and these options change over time. Other therapies can be recorded using the "Other" field and associated narrative box. Documenting the type of therapy used may have implications in terms of operative difficulty, postoperative recovery, and complications as well as lymph node retrieval and oncologic outcomes. Finally, it is important to assess the tumor's response to preoperative therapy.

**Note J:** Intraoperative Primary Tumor Findings, T Category

**Explanatory Comments:** In the context of this protocol for cancer surgery documentation, TNM categories from the American Joint Committee on Cancer (AJCC) are not designated with clinical (lower case "c" prefix) nor pathological (lower case "p" prefix) classifications. Determination of pathological classification involves a synthesis of information from multiple sources including clinical staging, operative findings, and pathological evaluation of resected surgical specimen(s). Complete information on TNM categories, clinical/pathological classifications, and the overall process of cancer staging can be found in the *AJCC Cancer Staging Manual,* Eighth Edition.

Thus, this field is to document the intraoperative findings pertaining to whether the primary tumor is confined to the stomach or not (T4a or T4b) as this helps inform pathological classification (see Table 2).

**Table 2.** Definition of Primary Tumor (T)

| T Category | T Criteria |
|---|---|
| TX | Primary tumor cannot be assessed |
| T0 | No evidence of primary tumor |
| Tis | Carcinoma *in situ*: intraepithelial tumor without invasion of the lamina propria, high-grade dysplasia |
| T1 | Tumor invades the lamina propria, muscularis mucosae, or submucosa |
| T1a | Tumor invades the lamina propria or muscularis mucosae |
| T1b | Tumor invades the submucosa |
| T2 | Tumor invades the muscularis propria* |
| T3 | Tumor penetrates the subserosal connective tissue without invasion of the visceral peritoneum or adjacent structures**, *** |
| T4 | Tumor invades the serosa (visceral peritoneum) or adjacent structures**, *** |
| T4a | Tumor invades the serosa (visceral peritoneum) |
| T4b | Tumor invades adjacent structures/organs |

* A tumor may penetrate the muscularis propria with extension into the gastrocolic or gastrohepatic ligaments, or into the greater or lesser omentum, without perforation of the visceral peritoneum covering these structures. In this case, the tumor is classified as T3. If there is perforation of the visceral peritoneum covering the gastric ligaments or the omentum, the tumor should be classified as T4.
** The adjacent structures of the stomach include the spleen, transverse colon, liver, diaphragm, pancreas, abdominal wall, adrenal gland, kidney, small intestine, and retroperitoneum.
*** Intramural extension to the duodenum or esophagus is not considered invasion of an adjacent structure, but is classified using the depth of the greatest invasion in any of these sites.

**Note K:** Intraoperative Lymph Node Findings, N Category

**Explanatory Comments:** In the context of this protocol for cancer surgery documentation, TNM categories from the AJCC are not designated with clinical (lower case "c" prefix) nor pathological (lower case "p" prefix) classifications. Determination of pathological classification involves a synthesis of information from multiple sources including clinical staging, operative findings, and pathological evaluation of resected surgical specimen(s). Complete information on TNM categories, clinical/pathological classifications, and the overall process of cancer staging can be found in the *AJCC Cancer Staging Manual,* Eighth Edition.

The presence and extent of regional lymphadenopathy is one of the most important prognostic features in gastric adenocarcinoma. This field documents the intraoperative findings pertaining to regional lymphadenopathy as this helps inform pathological staging (see Table 3). Adequate pathological staging of the regional lymph nodes is important and thus, a D2 lymphadenectomy is recommended. Therefore, if "suspected regional adenopathy" is selected, the surgeon is asked to answer whether the suspected regional adenopathy was completely resected or not. Information on non-regional or distant lymphadenopathy should be documented under Intraoperative Metastatic findings, M Category.

**Table 3.** Definition of Regional Lymph Node (N)

| N Category | N Criteria |
|---|---|
| NX | Regional lymph nodes cannot be assessed |
| N0 | No regional lymph node metastases |
| N1 | Metastasis in one to two regional lymph nodes |
| N2 | Metastasis in three to six regional lymph nodes |
| N3 | Metastasis in seven or more regional lymph nodes |
| N3a | Metastasis in seven to 15 regional lymph nodes |
| N3b | Metastasis in 16 or more regional lymph nodes |

**Note L:** Interoperative Metastatic Findings, M Category

**Explanatory Comments:** In the context of this protocol for cancer surgery documentation, TNM categories from the AJCC are not designated with clinical (lower case "c" prefix) nor pathological (lower case "p" prefix) classifications. Determination of pathological classification involves a synthesis of information from multiple sources including clinical staging, operative findings, and pathological evaluation of resected surgical specimen(s). Complete information on TNM categories, clinical/pathological classifications, and the overall process of cancer staging can be found in the *AJCC Cancer Staging Manual,* Eighth Edition.

Metastasis from gastric cancer can often be occult on staging imaging. Surgical staging is critical to identifying these radiographic occult metastases and has significant implications for treatment decisions and patient outcomes. Thus, this field is to document the intraoperative findings of peritoneal metastasis, distant lymphadenopathy, liver metastasis or ovarian (Kruckenberg) metastasis. Other sites of metastatic disease can be recorded using the "Other" field and associated narrative box. These findings help inform the pathological classification (see Table 4).

**Table 4.** Definition of Distant Metastasis (M)

| M Category | M Criteria (Exocrine Pancreas) |
|---|---|
| M0 | No distant metastasis |
| M1 | Distant metastasis |

**Note M:** Type of Resection

**Explanatory Comments:** The extent of gastric resection should be described clearly (see Table 5). Options are provided for types of gastrectomy, which include both anatomic and non-anatomic resections. Characterization of the amount of organ removed provides information that is pertinent to primary tumor location and extent, remaining stomach volume (if any), and type of reconstruction (if any). Total gastrectomy would include resection of the anatomic and histologic gastroesophageal junction along with the pylorus. Gastrectomy not otherwise specified (NOS), or terms like "partial" gastrectomy, should be avoided. A "near-total" and "subtotal" gastrectomy may be interpreted uniquely. A general recommendation is that cancers of the distal third of the stomach would receive a "distal gastrectomy," middle third of stomach lesions a "hemi- or subtotal gastrectomy," and tumors of the proximal third a "total gastrectomy."

**Table 5.** Relevant NCDB Site-Specific Surgery Codes for Stomach Adapted from *STORE* Manual

| NCDB Code | Definition |
|---|---|
| A300 | Gastrectomy, NOS (partial, subtotal, hemi-) |
| A310 | Antrectomy, lower (distal-less than 40% of stomach)*** |
| A320 | Lower (distal) gastrectomy (partial, subtotal, hemi-) |
| A330 | Upper (proximal) gastrectomy (partial, subtotal, hemi-) |
| A400 | Near-total or total gastrectomy, NOS |
| A410 | Near-total gastrectomy |
| A420 | Total gastrectomy |
| A500 | Gastrectomy, NOS WITH removal of a portion of esophagus |
| A510 | Partial or subtotal gastrectomy |
| A520 | Near total or total gastrectomy |
| A600 | Gastrectomy with a resection in continuity with the resection of other organs, NOS*** |
| A610 | Partial or subtotal gastrectomy, in continuity with the resection of other organs*** |
| A620 | Near total or total gastrectomy, in continuity with the resection of other organs*** |
| A630 | Radical gastrectomy, in continuity with the resection of other organs*** |
| A800 | Gastrectomy, NOS |

*** Incidental splenectomy NOT included

ACS Standards for *Oncology Registry Entry* (*STORE*) 2023. Appendix A: Site-Specific Surgery Codes, Stomach.

**Note N:** Omentectomy

**Explanatory Comments:** Important technical aspects of gastrectomy include removal of the greater and lesser omentum. The rationale for omentectomy is that occult metastasis may be found in the omentum, which is important for adequate pathologic staging. A complete greater omentectomy is typically performed during total gastrectomy, whereas a partial removal of the greater omentum associated with subtotal or distal gastrectomy is common. Ligation of the left gastric artery pedicle along with the lesser omentum is required for total gastrectomy. However, this may be performed selectively for distal gastrectomy.

**Note O:** Lymph Node Dissection

**Explanatory Comments:** Lymphadenectomy is a critical component of radical gastrectomy and is necessary for complete pathologic staging. A D0 lymph node dissection implies that a wedge (non-anatomic) resection of the stomach was performed without retrieval of any perigastric lymph nodes, or anything less than a D1 lymphadenectomy. D1 lymphadenectomy refers to the perigastric lymph nodes contained within the tissue immediately adjacent to (or contiguous with) the stomach. For a total gastrectomy, a D1 lymphadenectomy would include lymph node stations 1–7 (see gastric section of *Operative Standards for Cancer Surgery* Volume 2, pages 106-114). Because a D1 lymph node dissection would likely yield less than the 16 lymph nodes recommended for adequate staging, a D2 lymph node is required to yield sufficient nodes to align with the principles of staging. For a total gastrectomy, D2 lymphadenectomy includes D1 plus stations 8a, 9, 10, 11p, 11d, and 12a. These are lymph nodes anterior to the hepatoduodenal ligament nodes along the proper hepatic artery, anterior common hepatic artery, celiac trunk nodes, nodes along the splenic artery and the splenic hilum. A D3 lymphadenectomy is not considered in the operative standards.

**Note P:** Lymph Node Stations Harvested

**Explanatory Comments:** Attribution of the extent of lymphadenectomy (e.g., D1 vs. D2) requires an understanding of the individual lymph node stations. Lymph node stations 1–7 would be considered part of a D1 lymph node dissection commonly performed in a total gastrectomy. The addition of stations 8–12 constitutes a D2 lymphadenectomy for a total gastrectomy and would be most likely to generate the minimum number of lymph nodes (16) necessary for accurate pathologic staging.

 

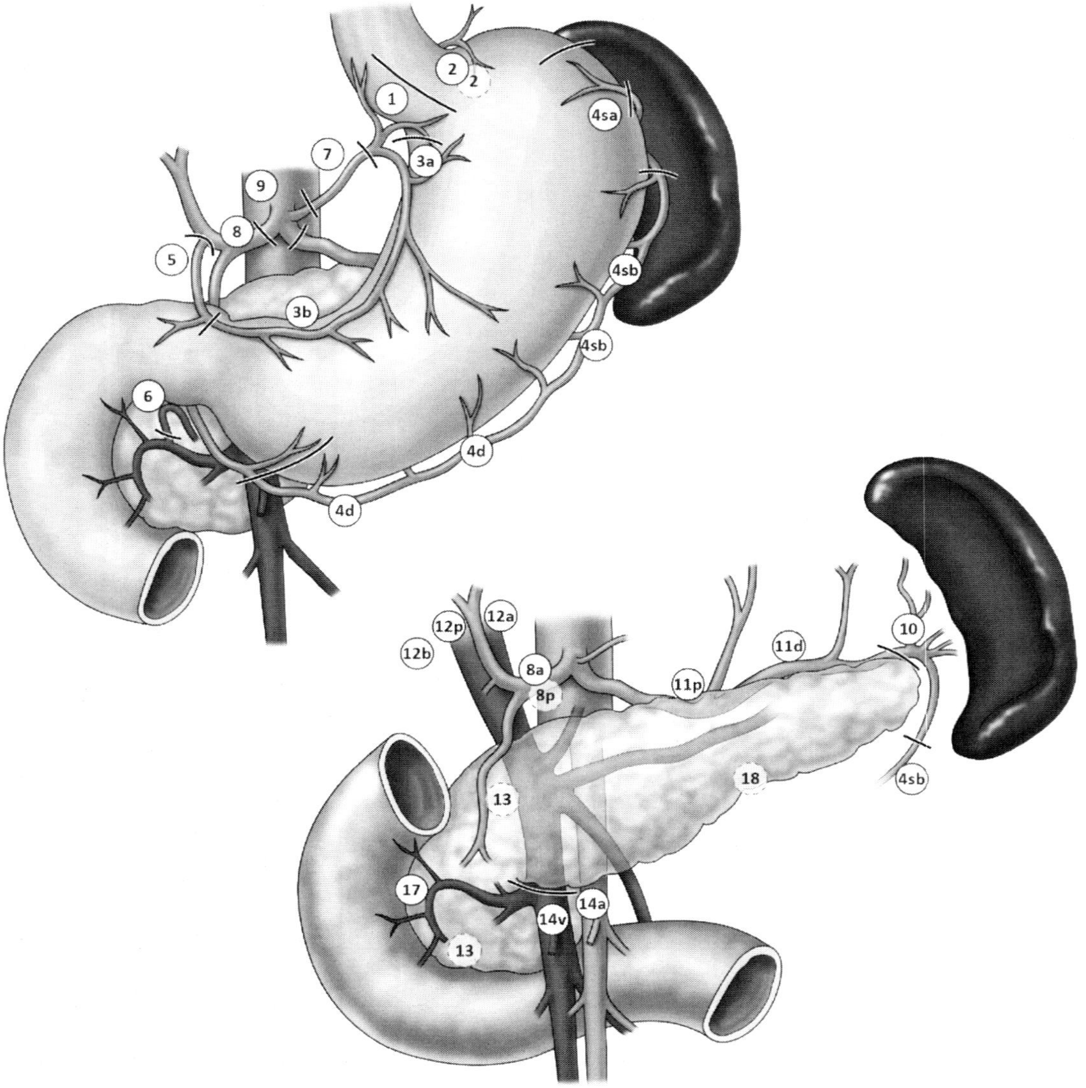


**Figure 1.** Location of lymph node stations based on the Japanese classification of gastric cancer. Adapted from the Japanese classification of gastric carcinoma: 3rd English edition. Gastric Cancer 2011 with permission.

**Table 6.** Lymph Node Stations for Figure 1

| Number | Definition |
|---|---|
| 1 | Right paracardial LNs, including those along the first branch of the ascending limb of the left gastric artery |
| 2 | Left paracardial LNs including those along the esophagocardiac branch of the left subphrenic artery |
| 3a | Lesser curvature LNs along the branches of the left gastric artery |
| 3b | Lesser curvature LNs along the second branch and distal part of the right gastric artery |
| 4sa | Left greater curvature LNs along the short gastric arteries (perigastric area) |
| 4sb | Left greater curvature LNs along the left gastroepiploic artery (perigastric area) |
| 4d | Right greater curvature LNs along the second branch and distal part of the right gastroepiploic artery |
| 5 | Suprapyloric LNs along the first branch and proximal part of the right gastric artery |
| 6 | Infrapyloric LNs along the first branch and proximal part of the right gastroepiploic artery down to the confluence of the right gastroepiploic vein and the anterior superior pancreatoduodenal vein |
| 7 | LNs along the trunk of left gastric artery between its root and the origin of its ascending branch |
| 8a | Anterosuperior LNs along the CHA |
| 8p | Posterior LNs along the CHA |
| 9 | Celiac artery LNs |
| 10 | Splenic hilar LNs including those adjacent to the splenic artery distal to the pancreatic tail, and those on the roots of the short gastric arteries and those along the left gastroepiploic artery proximal to its first gastric branch |
| 11p | Proximal splenic artery LNs from its origin to halfway between its origin and the pancreatic tail end |
| 11d | Distal splenic artery LNs from halfway between its origin and the pancreatic tail end to the end of the pancreatic tail |
| 12a | Hepatoduodenal ligament LNs along the proper hepatic artery, in the caudal half between the confluence of the right and left hepatic ducts and the upper border of the pancreas |
| 12b | Hepatoduodenal ligament LNs along the bile duct, in the caudal half between the confluence of the right and left hepatic ducts and the upper border of the pancreas |
| 12p | Hepatoduodenal ligament LNs along the portal vein in the caudal half between the confluence of the right and left hepatic ducts and the upper border of the pancreas |
| 13 | LNs on the posterior surface of the pancreatic head cranial to the duodenal papilla |
| 14v | LNs along the SMV |
| 15 | LNs along the middle colic vessels |
| 16a1 | Para-aortic LNs in the diaphragmatic aortic hiatus |
| 16a2 | Para-aortic LNs between the upper margin of the origin of the celiac artery and the lower border of the left renal vein |
| 16b1 | Para-aortic LNs between the lower border of the left renal vein and the upper border of the origin of the inferior mesenteric artery |
| 16b2 | Para-aortic LNs between the upper border of the origin of the inferior mesenteric artery and the aortic bifurcation |
| 17 | LNs on the anterior surface of the pancreatic head beneath the pancreatic sheath |
| 18 | LNs along the inferior border of the pancreatic body |
| 19 | Infradiaphragmatic LNs predominantly along the subphrenic artery |
| 20 | Paraesophageal LNs in the diaphragmatic esophageal hiatus |
| 110 | Paraesophageal LNs in the lower thorax |
| 111 | Supradiaphragmatic LNs separate from the esophagus |
| 112 | Posterior mediastinal LNs separate from the esophagus and the esophageal hiatus |

LN, lymph node; CHA, common hepatic artery; SMV, superior mesenteric vein. Source: Adapted from Japanese Gastric Cancer Association. Japanese classification of gastric carcinoma: 3rd English edition. Gastric Cancer 2011;14:101–112 (Table 5), 21 with permission.

**Note Q:** Margins

**Explanatory Comments:** Assessment of resection margins aims to increase the probability of a complete (R0) resection. Furthermore, an intraoperative margin assessment can inform the operating surgeon of not only the extent of resection, but also of tumor biology and oncologic benefit of R1 versus R0 resection (see gastric section of *Operative Standards for Cancer Surgery*, Volume 2, pages 100-106.

**Note R:** Completeness of Gastric Resection

**Explanatory Comments:** Documentation of residual gross disease is an important component of the operative report, given that only the surgeon can reliably distinguish an R1 margin from an R2 margin. R0/R1 should be indicated for cases when no gross tumor was left behind, irrespective of microscopic confirmation. An R2 response should be selected if there was macroscopic residual tumor, and a narrative box is provided to record additional details. Definitions for R Designation from the AJCC are summarized in Table 6. For additional details, please refer to the *Operative Standards for Cancer Surgery*, Volume 2, pages 100-106

**Table 7.** Definition of R Designation (Residual Tumor After Treatment)

| R | R Definition |
|---|---|
| R0 | No residual tumor |
| R1 | Microscopic residual tumor |
| R2 | Macroscopic residual tumor at the primary cancer site or regional nodal sites (This designation is not used to indicate metastatic disease identified but not resected at surgical exploration.) |

*AJCC Cancer Staging Manual*, Eighth Edition, Chapter 1 (Principles of Cancer Staging).

**Note S:** Adjacent Organs Resected

**Explanatory Comments:** Whether to perform additional surgeries should be individualized based on risks and benefits, and those details can be documented. In order to remove the tumor with negative margins, adjacent organs may be removed, or additional procedures may be performed at the surgeon's discretion in the management of the patient's cancer. Details can be recorded in the narrative box, as needed.

## Section 3: Additional Procedure Details

**Note T:** Operative Approach

**Explanatory Comments:** Several technical approaches to gastrectomy are now available for the surgical removal of the primary tumor and regional lymph nodes, including minimally invasive and open laparotomy procedures. Selection of the approach may be based on the patient and surgeon preference or other clinical factors. Use the narrative box to explain any circumstances outside of the options provided. Relevant NCDB codes are provided in Table 8 for the *Approach –Surgery of the Primary Site at this Facility (RxHospSurgApp 2010)* [668] data item from *STORE 2023*.

 

**Table 8.** Relevant NCDB Codes for *Approach – Surgery of the Primary Site at this Facility* from *STORE* Manual

| NCDB Code | Label |
|---|---|
| 0 | No surgical procedure of primary site at this facility; Diagnosed at autopsy |
| 1 | Robotic assisted |
| 2 | Robotic converted to open |
| 3 | Minimally invasive (such as endoscopic or laparoscopic) |
| 4 | Minimally invasive (endoscopic or laparoscopic) converted to open |
| 5 | Open or approach unspecified |

ACS *Standards for Oncology Registry Entry (STORE) 2023*. Approach–Surgery of the Primary Site at this Facility (RxHospSurgApp 2010).

*This table has been amended to remove code 9 (Unknown whether the surgery was performed at this facility) as it would not be an appropriate code in the context of this report.

**Note U:** Reconstruction Approach

**Explanatory Comments**: Following resection, the surgeon has a range of options for reconstruction. Please indicate whether the reconstruction was intracorporeal, extracorporeal, or used a mini-laparotomy.

**Note V:** Reconstruction Method

**Explanatory Comments:** Following gastric resection, the surgeon has a range of options for reconstruction. Please indicate whether a Bilroth II, Roux-en-Y, or Other reconstruction method was performed. If another reconstruction method was used, please use the narrative box to explain the details of the reconstruction.

**Note W:** Type of Esophago-jejunostomy

**Explanatory Comments:** Please indicate the method used to perform the anastomosis as Stapled (linear or circular stapler), Handsewn, or Other. If another method was used, please explain the details of the anastomosis. Technical details about the procedure can be entered in the narrative box, as needed.

**Note X:** Type of Gastro-Jejunostomy

**Explanatory Comments:** Please indicate the method used to perform the anastomosis as Stapled (linear or circular stapler), Handsewn, or Other. If another method was used, please explain the details of the anastomosis. Technical details about the procedure can be entered in the narrative box, as needed.

**Note Y:** Management of Duodenal 'Stump'

**Explanatory Comments:** The distal transection required to remove the stomach commonly occurs just distal to the pylorus in the first portion of the duodenum. The duodenal stump refers to the remaining part of the duodenum after transection. The transection and closure of the duodenum can be performed in various ways, often with the use of a stapling device. The cut-edge of the staple line can be reinforced with bioabsorbable materials, oversewing of the staple line, or both. Please indicate whether a stapler was used to divide and close to the duodenum or if another method was used. If stapled, indicate whether enforcement with bioabsorbable materials, oversewing of the staple line, or both were performed. Provide any additional detail about the procedure in the narrative box, as needed.

 

**Note Z:** Drains

**Explanatory Comments:** Surgical drains can be placed at the time of surgery for a variety of reasons. Please indicate whether a surgical drain was used and enter additional details about drain type, location, etc. in the narrative box, as needed.

**Note AA:** Feeding Tube

**Explanatory Comments:** Feeding tubes can be placed at the time of surgery to provide nutritional support. Please indicate whether a feeding tube was placed and enter additional details about feeding tube type, location, etc. in the narrative box, as needed.

**Note AB:** Additional Procedures

**Explanatory Comments:** Whether to perform additional surgeries should be individualized based on risk and benefits, and those details can be documented here. Similarly, adjacent organs may be removed, or additional procedures may be performed at the surgeon's discretion in the management of the patient's cancer. Details can be recorded in the narrative box, as needed.

**Note AC:** Additional Surgical Variables

**Explanatory Comments:** While concordance with operative standards has been the primary focus of this SOR, end user focus groups requested the scope of the tool to be expanded in order for it to comply with all surgical reporting requirements. As a result, this report can now be considered a comprehensive operative report, and it can be used to help generate billing codes and output data into hospital registries. There was not sufficient consensus, however, on non-cancer surgical information, such as patient positioning, incision location, port placement, fascial closure, etc., and so narrative text options are provided for inserting information the surgeon considers important.

**Note AD:** Intraoperative Complications

**Explanatory Comments:** Intraoperative complications are rare, but important to document them regardless of whether they are related to focal surgical difficulties or systemic events that may relate to patient positioning, delivery of anesthesia, or other aspects of the surgical procedure.

## References

1. Ajani JA, D'Amico TA, Bentrem DJ, et al. Gastric Cancer, Version 2.2022, NCCN Clinical Practice Guidelines in Oncology. Journal of the National Comprehensive Cancer Network; 2022.
2. Amin MB, Edge SB, Greene FL, et al, eds. *AJCC Cancer Staging Manual*. 8th ed. New York, NY: Springer; 2017.
3. Commission on Cancer. *Standards for Oncology Registry Entry (STORE)*. Chicago, IL: American College of Surgeons; 2023.
4. Hunt KK, Katz MH, Veeramachaneni N, et al. *Operative Standards for Cancer Surgery*. Vol 2. Chicago, IL: Wolters Kluwer; 2019.
5. Japanese classification of gastric carcinoma: 3rd English edition. Gastric Cancer; 2011.

 

Made in United States
North Haven, CT
05 November 2026

21767748R00015